MAKE TIME FOR YOURSELF

A more relaxed you is a more productive you!

Written by Raphaëlle Julie H.

Translated by Ciaran Traynor

Health and Wellbeing 50MINUTES.com

MAKE TIME FOR YOURSELF

- **Problem**: between work, friends, family, grocery shopping and cooking, trying to fit everything into our hectic modern lives is not easy. But where does our precious time go? How can we reconnect with what we really want and need?
- **Aims**: to become aware of how to take care of yourself and your time and learn to manage your life more calmly with the help of a few simple tricks.
- **FAQs**:
    - What does making time for yourself mean?
    - Why is it so difficult to make time for myself?
    - How can I allow myself to put my own wellbeing before that of others every now and then ?
    - How can I differentiate between what is good for me and what holds me back?
    - How can I organise myself and give myself the time I need to feel calm in my everyday life?
    - How can I stay in touch with who I really am?

Do you give yourself some alone time every now and then, a time for you to recharge your batteries and listen to yourself? Do you see life as a succession of happy events or a mountain of responsibilities you have to face up to?

When you want to harmonise your career with your family life, your social life with your exercise regime, or your artistic life with your beliefs, you may not really know what to do. The desire to match up to a certain image or find fulfilment while still carrying out our duties pushes us to accept situations in which we no longer respect who we really are. We forget to take care of our bodies and ignore our mental health. We may sometimes even feel like robots. Once we become prisoners of this system, we lose sight of the doors to freedom.

Although life is precious, it can exhaust us just as easily as it can invigorate us. Everything depends on how we live and how we manage our relationships with others, our environment and ourselves. Becoming aware of how we organise our days, our activities and our moments of rest is the first step. The second is to learn to listen to our greatest needs and desires. Although this requires a little imagination, organisation or even a certain ability to let go, it is possible to make time for yourself in order to live a balanced, fulfilling life. We only have one life – it would be a shame to waste it!

WHY IS IT DIFFICULT TO MAKE TIME FOR YOURSELF?

THE 21ST-CENTURY ILLNESS – LACK OF TIME

In the past, our ancestors lived according to the rhythm of the seasons and nature. Nowadays, ever since the Industrial Revolution, machines facilitate our manual, household and administrative work. However, our quality of life does not really seem to have improved. Caught in a vicious circle, we no longer have the time to stop to take a breath, or even to live our lives! We feel caught up in an eternal whirlwind, in a world where everything goes too fast.

Consequently, it is more and more difficult for us to catch our breath in a society in which we have to take on more and more demands, information and requests. The media overwhelm us on a daily basis with images, each more depressing than the last. The future does not look promising, with unemployment, violence and environmental problems all on the rise. However, as Marcelle Auclair (French author, 1899-1983) states in *Le Livre du bonheur* ("The Book of Happiness"), joy, love and happiness truly do exist. It is up to us to decide whether we want to focus on the misery in the world or, on the contrary, to adopt a positive view of life. However, is it possible that we still do not have all the keys to unlock the door to happiness?

Together, we will look at the way you give yourself time to be in harmony with yourself. We will then analyse the traps which prevent you from correctly dividing up your different responsibilities. Finally, we will look at the idea of enjoyment, which should be a central part of life. However, being able to experience this type of feeling in our daily lives is not as evident as it may seem, since we are so disconnected from the present. In order to achieve this we need time to focus on the essential and on ourselves. We have to give ourselves the position we deserve in our lives. However, if we want to live more freely, the first thing we need to do is to find out how we function.

TIME FOR SOME SELF-EXAMINATION!

Begin by buying a notebook which takes your fancy. Choose the colour, the format and the material, and write "Time for myself" in big letters on the front cover. Every morning, open it up, grab a pen and get writing! For example, write down how you feel when you wake up: are you happy to get up and looking forward to experiencing new things? Or, on the contrary, do you already feel tired thinking about all the tasks waiting for you?

WHERE DOES THE TIME GO?

The Tale of Eve and the Land of Dreams
The city of love, salty-sweet treats, multicoloured masks....
Venice really has it all! Eve dreams of taking her boyfriend there. But each time she tries to book the romantic weekend away, something comes up. And so she just keeps putting the dream off for another day.

If you ask Eve why she never gets around to booking her city trip, she will tell you that she never has the time: her best friend would call her mid-crisis, her mum was in the middle of moving or her boss had just given her a new file to work on. She feels she cannot manage her time any more. She feels constantly overwhelmed by what Alec MacKenzie, an American researcher and author of the famous book *The Time Trap: The Classic Book on Time Management*, likes to call "time traps". These "time traps" are all the elements which slowly chip away at both your professional and private organisation.

Alec MacKenzie classifies these distractions into two categories:

- **External traps**: external elements which disturb what you are doing or your organisation. For example, phones, social media, meetings and business lunches are particularly good examples of this type of trap.
- **Internal traps**, such as lack of organisation, inability to delegate, perfectionism, bad time management, and so on.

Although external time-wasting factors are easy to detect, internal causes are more insidious. It is therefore important to analyse your behaviour to detect the elements which take up a lot of your day.

Internal traps	External traps
....	....
....	....
....	....
....	....
....	....
....	....
....	....
....	....
....	....
....	....
....	

LACK OF ORGANISATION

Organisation is a personal and subjective ability. It varies according to an individual's personality, education or background. Although it is not the easiest thing to master, you should still learn to organise yourself if you want to change your bad habits. Indeed, better use of your time will allow you to accomplish your everyday tasks while still allowing yourself moments of rest, which are essential for good mental and physical balance.

ARE YOU ORGANISED?

To find out if you are an organised person, answer the following questions:

- Is your desk tidy? Are your papers filed? Is everything in order?

- Do you use plans, diagrams or lists to organise your work?
- Is your house pleasant to live in? Easy to keep clean? Does everyone who lives there take part in household tasks? Do you know how to delegate?
- Do you respect your limits? Do you, for example, take power naps, the short siestas which are highly valued in the world of work for their restorative powers?

BEING AFRAID OF TAKING YOUR TIME

The Tortoise or the Tale of Little Rose
There was once a little tortoise called Rose who walked too slowly. Her friends and family would constantly tell her to "hurry up, hurry up!" One day, she decided to go more quickly, but she has been sad ever since.

While you were still just a child, you learned to do everything quickly. Both at school and at home, you had to adapt to the general rhythm. While speed was obviously seen as a good thing, taking your time, on the other hand, could be perceived as a sign of laziness or even as a lack of vitality. However, children all have their personal rhythm. If this rhythm is respected, they will pour their heart into everything they do. They all have many talents. The important thing to do is to let them develop without rushing them.

WHAT ABOUT YOU?

Did you feel free to live according to your own rhythm when you were a child? Were you overwhelmed with activities and demands?

If put in a similar situation to Rose, the majority of us would also begin to speed up. But at what cost? We cannot deny depression, burnout and other failings in communication. These syndromes often appear later on and are mostly due to the pushing away of our real needs.

If we are not allowed to live according to our own rhythm, we become trapped in a system where we forget to laugh, dream and make the most of life. And what if children are right? What if taking your time to do things with love is the key to happiness? If we have never been given this permission, will we give it to ourselves today?

THE DIFFICULTY OF ALLOWING YOURSELF TO PUT YOUR OWN WELLBEING BEFORE THAT OF OTHERS

We have almost all learned to put others before ourselves. And when we need to take some time for ourselves, we feel selfish. We experience this feeling of guilt mostly because of modern society, which encourages us to view this essential need as selfishness or indifference. However, how can we give others what they need if we feel empty?

One evening, take some time to write in your notebook. Choose a place that you love: your room, your conservatory, or simply a tree that you like sitting under.

Think about your day and try to differentiate between what you did for others and what you did for yourself.

For others	For myself

Where do you put your work? What about the time you spend with your children?

After analysing your answers, write down and complete this sentence "Today, I enjoyed..." This will help you to highlight elements that you took something positive out of, even if they were done for someone else.

LACK OF AWARENESS OF YOURSELF AND YOUR ENVIRONMENT

Where are you Tristan?
"That guy's as high as a kite!"
"No he's not! He's just a dreamer."
This is the story of a mysterious lad who wanders the streets and shelters under bridges. The years go by, and his beard gets longer. One day, a bird flies down onto his shoulder and sings him its song. He shivers. Suddenly, his voice and the songs he used to know come flooding back to him. And that's how our lad came to sing at the opera!

A concept made famous by the Belgian sociologist Marcel Bolle de Bal (born in 1930), "reliance" is the act of being connected to yourself while still being linked to your surroundings. In a way, it is about reaching a kind of global conscience of your being and environment and anchoring yourself firmly in reality. Reliance involves the individual being physically and mentally present in everything that they do. Have you ever noticed that a distracted person seems to be completely removed from the situation, and sometimes seems to not even be there at all? How can you take part in your own life if there is something missing? Being present means being well-anchored in the world, living in your body and using your feelings and your intuition to understand the world around you.

However, in a society where rational intelligence is king, are we still aware of our physical feelings? Of our emotions? Of our intuition? Our link to the world begins to fray when we are running about nonstop and forget to breathe. Without this reliance, we lose our connection with the universe, risk simply doing instead of being, and are in danger of just functioning instead of taking part. As the Belgian author Colette Nys-Mazure (born in 1939) explains:

> "What wears us down is not the constant recurrence of words and gestures or the inescapable return of seasons, but rather it is our absence from the flow of events, our lack of participation in the unceasing miracle [life]." (Colette Nys-Mazure, 2004: 16.)

QUICK-FIRE ROUND

Answer these questions right now, without over-thinking them:

- Do you pay attention to your feelings?
- What are the smells, the images and the noises around you at this precise moment? Describe them. What do you feel?

What about your emotions? As the Belgian author Marie-Pascale Coenraets so poetically puts it, emotions are to the soul what blood is to the body. They are responsible for you opening yourself to or shutting yourself away from life. But, in that case, why should you be afraid? If you accept them and think about what they mean for you, they will become excellent guides. However, if you repress them, they may take over your life and begin to wear you down. Will you still be able to understand them when they come crashing down on you like a tsunami?

Answer these questions right now, without over-thinking them:

- What are you feeling, right now? Are you at peace? Are you overwhelmed by an emotion? If so, which? What colour would it be? Do you know what it is linked to?
- Are you in the habit of expressing your feelings? Can you share what you have gone through with others? Do you feel that you are understood?

FINDING THE TIME TO LIVE

A STEP-BY-STEP PROGRAMME

Is learning to sit yourself down and get organised too difficult? Do your habits seem impossible to shake off? Although this is quite normal, this kind of habit should not prevent you from enjoying life and making time for yourself, as long as you set yourself realistic objectives, of course... And go about them step by step!

Jane is the mother of a sick little boy. She has been looking after him for two years night, day and night, with an endless stream of love.

> "I get help. My partner is really great! But I just couldn't find the time to catch my breath. So I decided to meet a counsellor. Seeing how tired I was – particularly mentally – she suggested that I stop everything for three minutes every day. Three minutes doesn't seem like much. But I just couldn't do it! We then moved on to something that seemed more realistic to me: three seconds a day. Whenever I came out of the shower, I would stop for three seconds to breathe deeply. It was a start!
> I've now moved on to the next stage: each morning, in the lotus position, I allow myself ten minutes to breathe. I then calmly visualise my day. It doesn't seem like much, but it really puts me in the right frame of mind; I start the day far more relaxed!"

In order to regain lost time for yourself, you have to put in place foundations and persevere. You need to discipline yourself and force yourself to take time just for yourself. You heard right: force yourself! Like this young mother, who forced herself to give herself a few seconds of respite every day. Through hard work, she eventually managed to allow herself ten minutes a day to breathe and clear her mind. What an accomplishment!

Perseverance is also extremely important. As Daniel Sévigny, an author and thought management trainer from Quebec, highlights, our brain is conditioned by our beliefs and our experiences. Through repetition, our thoughts create neurocircuits. We have to repeat a new action for 21 days to break the circuits made by bad habits. Effective change takes time. Why not begin today by adopting a new behaviour or reciting a positive thought for three weeks to make a new habit?

EXERCISE

Invent a key phrase that you will recite like a mantra for 21 days. For example: "I know that life is full of happiness, and I'm going to find it" or "I listen to and follow my desires. I make the most of life!"

If the Buddhist monk Thich Nhat Hanh (born in 1926) is to be believed, being able to live in the moment is neither a quality nor a question of faith, but a question of practice!

So make the most of life, and never give up, no matter what happens! Other people have proved that it is worth the effort. Take Dominique Glocheux, for instance, who found himself paralysed after an accident. All he could do was move his finger. With nothing but this single finger, he wrote incredible books. His message? "Life is sweet!"[1] (Glocheux, 1998)

LEARNING TO BE ORGANISED

A structured living space

Sylvain is a writer. He works at home, a 60 m² apartment in Brussels that he shares with his wife and their two children. They ran out of room very quickly.

> "I ended up not being able to find what I'd written. When I looked after the children, I couldn't find their clothes or their toys. It was even worse in the kitchen – it was an absolute shambles. Finally, the untidiness became an obsession, and I couldn't focus on anything else. We didn't have the money to rent a bigger apartment, and I felt trapped.
> One day, a friend came by the house. We gathered everything up and sorted through it, and then either sold or gave away some items and bought furniture and boxes to tidy things away. Our nest became a whole lot cosier. We have fewer things now, but everything is there for a reason!"

To feel good at home, you have to organise your living space. Create a place that suits you and which you like. In order to do this, think about smells, materials and colours which you like.

---

1. This quotation has been translated by 50Minutes.com.

Do not forget the advantages of a good spring clean. In Japan, for example, New Year is a very important celebration. The festivities last several days and begin with *Oosoji*, a house-wide New-Year clean which the whole family takes part in.

Why not do the same? Get the family together, choose some encouraging music and get started! Clear the shelves, throw out all that rubbish in the loft, and scrub those floorboards! It will be an unforgettable experience, and a guaranteed success! Your little nest will be all the better for it.

Here are five pieces of advice to help you to stay organised:

- Sort through your things and sell whatever you no longer need to a second-hand shop or give it to charity.
- Invest in storage.
- Find the best place for each object. This will save you having to look for it when you need it.
- Always tidy up as you go along instead of leaving things to build up.
- Share tasks out between the different members of the household.

Organise your time

In the morning, plan your day in your diary. Write down your meetings, your obligations, and the wind-down time you are going to give yourself. Your timetable has got to be as realistic as possible, even if you have the feeling that you are drowning in work. Do not forget to give yourself time to re-charge your batteries. By organising yourself effectively, you will have time to breathe. You may have already managed this in the past. Do not forget that nobody is asking you to keep a rhythm where you are forced to run everywhere throughout the day to keep up. Check your diary regularly: it will be your guide.

Keep your evenings free for your passions and your weekends for your friends or children. Turn your computer and television off every now and then and try something new!

TIP

Here is some advice from Lisa: "I often leave blank slots in my schedule so I feel free to do what I want to!"

Mastering the time traps

Now that you know that time traps exist, have you been able to identify some external ones? Have you also detected the internal problems which are disrupting the flow of your time management? Peter Drucker (management expert, 1909-2005) proved that internal time traps are the real problem. In other words, outside invaders manage to break into your life because you let them!

Take for example a company boss who is always late. He complains that he has to do all his employees' work, which distracts him from his real objectives. He has the feeling that he never gets anything finished. One by one, his clients begin to complain. If this man analyses his situation, he will realise that the problem is not his employees, but him, because he simply cannot delegate. By trying to control everything, he no longer controls anything!

To get rid of your internal traps, you have to be able to identify them. When a situation becomes a problem, the best thing to do is to take a step back to analyse the facts. You have to be able to question yourself. How has the situation ended up like this? What have you done to make things this way? What fears forced you to act in this way? If you are bothered by other people, give yourself some alone time. Think up strategies to be calm when you feel the need.

You also have to establish your limits so you do not accept everything suggested to you, to the point that you no longer have any time for yourself. To paraphrase Jean-Louis Servan-Schreiber (born in 1937), the author of *The Art of Time*, mastering your time means mastering yourself.

Follow your own rhythm and enjoy life

The first thing to do is to get to know your essential needs by answering these few questions:

- How many hours of sleep do you need to feel in optimal

form?
- What is your natural rhythm? Are you more effective in the morning or at night?
- Do you enjoy strolling down streets or going running in the park to let off steam?
- What gives you more energy: naps or dancing?
- What makes you nervous? Unhappy?
- On the other hand, what does you good and what makes you happy?

When you realise that you can slow down, a world of possibilities will open up to you! You can, for example, get back into cooking, gardening, learning a language, and so on. Basically, you can do all those things that you wanted to do but never had time for.

Do not feel guilty about taking pleasure in things and giving yourself time to dream. Life is a gift. Happiness can often be found in the simple things in life. Watch a bird land, eat a slice of chocolate cake, dress up, go walking in the moonlight. All of these little moments open up our senses, calm us or fill us with joy.

Listen to what you really want and act accordingly! Do not ignore your body either: do you want to sleep, stay at home, run, cry, love, etc.? Do it. Listen to yourself. And congratulate yourself for doing so!

Madeleine was the happy mother of four children. But when they did not help her around the house, she would sometimes grab her keys, slam the door and go off in her car for an hour. It was her way of telling herself that this was the

last straw. Because Madeleine would do everything – sometimes even too much. So when she cracked, she definitely
cracked!

> "But one day, I discovered something that changed my life.
> I bought myself a *Hello* magazine and settled myself down
> with a coffee and a chocolate. Bliss!
> When I go for my *Hello* magazine break, everyone knows that
> I am not to be disturbed. This is my bubble, my me-time!"

Let yourself fantasise! Life is not a prison! On the contrary, it
is the perfect place to open yourself up, learn, grow and take
risks. Look at children – they learn by playing. Each day, they
play, laugh and experiment. Be like them and enjoy yourself
whenever you have the chance! "You don't need much to
be happy", "Happiness is a journey, not a destination" and
"Happiness is its own reward" are all expressions to remind
you that you too can be personally fulfilled, as long as you
let yourself.

IN YOUR NOTEBOOK

Write up everything you like doing. Why not take inspi-
ration from Julie Andrews' "My Favourite Things" from
The Sound of Music?

Think about yourself

In *Being Generous: The Art of Right Living*, Lucinda Vardey
and John Dalla Costa remind us of the need to be in harmony
with ourselves before giving time to others.

You need to look after yourself and know your needs and limits before being strong for someone else. If you do not prioritise yourself, you will have nothing to give others. It is obvious that a person who exhausts themselves and gives away all their energy without thinking about themselves ends up with nothing more to give. It is therefore important to focus on yourself and your essential needs to give yourself happiness and comfort. Most of all, you have to learn to respect yourself by setting limits and being able to say no.

We all have a little child inside us who is just begging to be coddled. Learn to listen to them and look after them. They are your link to joy, to your roots and to your real nature. For example, you can imagine yourself as a tree with roots firmly anchored in the ground; curl your inner child up right under your branches, sheltered from the elements.

Do not be afraid to set limits and say no

It is not always easy to say no, because we often fear that we will let people down. It is true that our generosity is appreciated when we help others. However, being able to establish limits is essential and beneficial to all relationships, whether they are social, professional or romantic. Being able to say no allows you to take control of your choices and, by extension, your time. Do not forget that the real gift is the one given freely and gladly.

No one will force you to justify a decision or a refusal, but if doing so will help you to be at peace with yourself, go for it! Express yourself clearly and calmly, and share what you feel.

Get back to basics

Before becoming a mother, Iris was – in her own words – a bulldozer. She would power through a huge amount of work every day, completely focused on what she had to do. When her little girl, Nina, was born, a feeling of urgency overcame Iris, and she felt that she had start looking at life differently. Since then, she has decided to reduce her working hours.

> "I didn't want to be a mother in name only. I learned to take the time to enjoy life. [...] Thanks to Nina, I discovered that pleasure can be found anywhere! My life no longer revolves around tasks and obligations. I believe that I have become more in touch with my senses. With Nina, I walk barefoot in the grass, I smell the clothes that I take out of the machine, and I've started learning how to do oil massages and self-massages. I even talk to my chickens!"

Thanks to the concept of reliance, you now know that it is important to be connected to yourself (your body, your experiences, your dreams), the world around you (nature, living beings) and time (your past and present). You should therefore listen to your:

- **Physical sensations**. Live and feel with your senses.
- **Emotions**. They are the colours of the passing time.
- **Your intuition**. Listen to this little inner voice. It knows what is right for you.

The essential is here and now. Your presence with yourself is what links you to everything. Little rituals can connect you to happiness: having a coffee with your neighbour every Saturday, admiring the sky with your partner every evening, lighting a candle during a simple meal, and so on.

A FEW METHODS TO HELP YOU

Certain techniques have been proven to be very effective in helping you to be more Zen and make the most of the present.

Zen Buddhism

The Buddhist practices of meditation and awakening, commonly practiced in Japan and China (although originally from India), are universally recognised for their benefits. Many scientists have demonstrated the advantage of meditation for the human brain: it brings a feeling of wholeness, better decision-making abilities, physical and psychological relaxation, and a feeling of self-presence.

Among these, zazen, which literally means "seated meditation", brings us to a state of non-waiting, of letting go. As Nicolas Gounaropoulos, who has been teaching this posture for 20 years, testifies:

> "By letting go, emotions like joy and compassion simply spring up. The whole art is allowing yourself to be influenced by this space within our conditioned experiences (work, family life)."[2] (Shi Deng Sangha)

Mindfulness

Mindfulness is a relaxation technique and way of connecting to yourself. Adapted to our cultures, this meditation is based on Vipassanā meditation. Breathing, mastering your mind, understanding your behaviour, getting to know yourself and, finally, breaking free of all the thoughts cluttering your mind are the different stages of this relaxation technique, which is one of the most ancient in India. 2500 years ago, it was the remedy to every ailment. Today, mindfulness is practiced in hospitals, where it has incredible results on patients with mental problems. This method is also very successful in schools and businesses.

Sophrology

Sophrology is a relaxation and visualisation method based on breathing. During sophrology sessions, a psychologist

---

2. This quotation has been translated by 50Minutes.com.

guides the learner with the help of self-calming techniques. The body exercises involved are quite simple. They teach you to get in touch with your feelings and accept them, and also help you to acquire tools which will be useful in everyday life.

IN FUTURE, DO NOT FORGET ABOUT YOURSELF!

Do not forget that, every day, you are the one who has control over your life. Taking time to develop yourself is neither a luxury nor a whim, but an absolute necessity!

A FEW FINAL TIPS

- Keep your diary updated and organise your days.
- Do not be afraid to say no and set limits.
- Learn to delegate and accept help when you need it.
- Take the time to breathe. If you feel overwhelmed by stress, tiredness or weariness, stop for a moment and breathe deeply.
- When you feel that you are losing control, take a step back and analyse the situation calmly.
- At the end of each day, look back over what you have done with the help of your notebook. Did you give yourself some time to enjoy yourself? Did you manage your tasks correctly?
- Do not forget that your outlook on life can change how you approach the day. Adopt a positive attitude.
- Pay attention to what you feel. The signals your body sends you help you to maintain your personal balance.

- Do not judge yourself and do not feel guilty about taking time for yourself.

FAQS

WHAT DOES MAKING TIME FOR YOURSELF MEAN?

"Time is money", as the saying goes. But what are we really chasing? Money, or the passing time?

In more concrete terms, making time for yourself means, for example, giving yourself a few minutes rest every day to breathe, begin a rewarding activity, or carry out a ritual which you enjoy. To put it simply, it helps you make the most of life.

Above all, should time not be a way to live in harmony with ourselves, our friends and family, and the world around us?

WHY IS IT SO DIFFICULT TO MAKE TIME FOR MYSELF?

There are several reasons which can prevent us from making the most of our time. Sometimes, we do not listen to our needs, our desires or our limits. At other times, we allow ourselves to be overwhelmed by "time traps" that we cannot identify. Sometimes, we do not correctly manage our time because of a lack of organisation. Finally, we may not let ourselves think about ourselves and make the most of good times.

HOW CAN I ALLOW MYSELF TO PUT MY OWN WELLBEING BEFORE THAT OF OTHERS EVERY NOW AND THEN?

Whether through kindness or timidity, some people just cannot say no and systematically put the needs of others before their own. They generally regret it, because this inability to set limits leads to a kind of suffering that often affects those around them.

It is therefore essential to realise that giving your time means listening to people and giving practical help and advice. It is a gift. And a gift should always be offered willingly and gladly.

HOW CAN I DIFFERENTIATE BETWEEN WHAT IS GOOD FOR ME AND WHAT HOLDS ME BACK?

To write up a list of all the things which help you to develop and those which prevent you from doing so, you have to take a step back and analyse how you are living. When you have distinguished the activities that give you pleasure from those which hold you back, you can grow as a person.

For example, you may feel overwhelmed by your possessions, in which case you need to sort through them, give away those you do not want and throw away those that you neither want to keep nor give away. If your relationships are a problem for you, take a look at how you impose your limits and how you act with your colleagues and those close to you. Can you say no? Do you feel guilty about allowing yourself to enjoy your own time?

Take the various situations you find yourself in and analyse them. What benefits can you get out of them? Which have become sources of stress and anxiety? Then imagine what steps you can take to remedy everything that disrupts your balance. Do not forget that you are often your own worst enemy.

According to Tibetan sages, a mind obsessed by the past does not allow us to make the most of the present. The same goes for uncertainties about the future. The past can cast new light on the present, just like envisioning the future can help you to make plans. But it is important to remember that certain obsessions are not constructive and will hold you back.

HOW CAN I ORGANISE MYSELF AND GIVE MYSELF THE TIME I NEED TO FEEL CALM IN MY EVERYDAY LIFE?

As soon as you stop giving yourself time, you withdraw from your own existence. Tiredness, nervousness and anxiety immediately appear and make you feel that you are no longer yourself.

Good organisation can help you to work efficiently, respect your natural rhythm and give yourself breaks to relax and think about yourself.

To help yourself do this, try to:

- observe the way you function,
- locate the most time-consuming parts of your day and try to control them,
- organise your day effectively,
- divide up daily tasks fairly,
- remember to take a step back every now and then,
- give yourself relaxation time,
- listen to what you want and respect your needs.

Taking some time to swim, do some DIY, go for a massage or even just read is absolutely essential. We have to allow ourselves to experience the joy of discovering, sharing and reconnecting with what makes us tick.

HOW CAN I STAY IN TOUCH WITH WHO I REALLY AM?

Scientists have proved that intuition truly does exist, as they found that there is an area of the brain which activates when we use it. As Dr David O'Hare explains in his book *Intuitions*, our inner voice can help us to make better decisions.

As a result, stay connected to what you want and pay attention to your needs. Be both the child who takes pleasure in what they are doing and the protective mother who looks after them.

Just be yourself and realise your dreams. "Dreams only disappear if you don't use them"[3] (Garagnon, 2001).

---

3. This quotation has been translated by 50Minutes.com.

We want to hear from you!
Leave a comment on your online library
and share your favourite books on social media!

FURTHER READING

BIBLIOGRAPHY

- Anselme, C. (2012) *Méditer transforme votre cerveau*. Bio info magazine, 118.
- Archimbaud, J. (No date) Jeannine Archimbaud, passeur d'histoires. *Lareliancecom*. [Online]. [Accessed 5 July 2017]. Available from: <http://www.lareliance.com/>
- Association-mindfulness.org. (No date) *Association pour le développement de la Mindfulness*. [Online]. [Accessed 5 July 2017]. Available from: <http://www.association-mindfulness.org/>
- Auclair, M. (2003) *Le livre du bonheur*. Paris: Seuil.
- Benoit, A. (2007) *La Zen Attitude des paresseuses*. Vanves: Éditions Marabout.
- De Biolley E. (No date) Everard de Biolley, praticien en PCI, sophrologue : Gestion de nos émotions au quotidien. *Gestion-emotion-quotidien.be*. [Online]. [Accessed 10 August 2015]. Available from: <http://www.gestion-emotion-quotidien.be/>
- Coenraets, M-P. (2012) *Et si j'ouvrais la porte de mon sixième sens ?* Wavre: Éditions Mols.
- Crawford, I. (1998) *La Maison du bien-être*. Paris: Armand Colin.
- Delhamende, M-A. (2007) Zen. *Agenda Plus*, 191.
- Garagnon, F. (2001) *Jade et les Sacrés Mystères de ma vie*. Épagny: Monte-Cristo Editions.
- Glocheux, D. (1998) *C'est doux la vie*. Paris: Éditions Flammarion.
- Glocheux, D. (1999) *Le Bonheur c'est les autres*. Paris:

Éditions Flammarion.
* Gounaropoulos, N. (No date) Shi Deng Sangha. *Shi Deng Sangha.be*. [Online]. [Accessed 12 August 2015]. Available from: <http://www.shidengsangha.be/>
* Hanh, T. N. (2009) *Le Sérénité de l'instant*. Paris: Éditions J'ai Lu.
* Hanh, T. N. (No date) Thich Nhat Hanh. *Thich-nhat-hanh. fr* [Online]. [Accessed 12 August 2015]. Available from: <http://www.thich-nhat-hanh.fr/>
* Lenoir, F. (2010) Petit traité de vie intérieure. Paris: Plon.
* Nys-Mazure, C. (2004) *Celebration of the Everyday*. Trans. Renée Linkhorn. New York: Peter Lang.
* O'Hare, D. and Phild, J-M. (2011) *Intuitions*. Vergèze: Thierry Souccar Éditions.
* Servan-Schreiber, J-L. (2000) *The Art of Time*. New York: Marlowe & Company.
* Singer, C. (2001) *Où cours-tu ? Ne sais-tu pas que le ciel est en toi ?* Paris: Albin Michel.
* Tolle, E. (2000) *Le Pouvoir du moment présent*. Outremont: Les Éditions Ariane.
* Vardey, L. and Dalla Costa, J. (2009) *Being Generous: The Art of Right Living*. Toronto: Vintage Canada.

ADDITIONAL SOURCES

* Keenan, K. (2015) *Make time: Learn How to Manage Your Time and Make More Time for Yourself*. Bath: Pocket Manager Books.

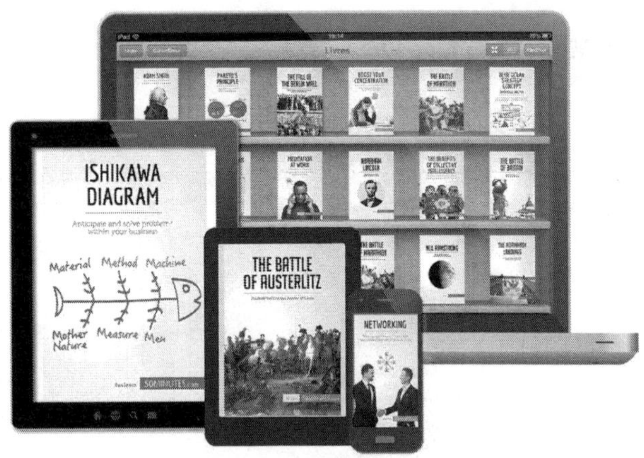

Made in the USA
Monee, IL
07 July 2026

56544697R00022